Eventually, we all must die. No one wants to think about it, but it is going to happen anyways. When it does, it can leave family or friends both sad and confused. Many times, there are things that were not important to you at all that become a big deal to your family. Or things that were important to you that your support system would have been happy to assist with, but was not discussed. Use this prompt journal to help you to think about all the things you want someone to know before you pass on. Then tell people about it, put it in a place they can find it, and be at peace that you gave this one last gift to those you love.

What were your Favorite Things in this lifetime?

What do you want people to remember about you?

What are your best memories?

What are you glad you did?

Where are you glad you went?

What are your biggest regrets?

What was the hardest thing you did?

What do you wish you could have done?

What is your best advice to those you leave behind?

How do you feel about your career?

What career do you wish you could have done?

What are your biggest accomplishments?

What are your favorite songs?

What is your favorite food?

What family recipes are your favorite?

What are your favorite movies?

What are your favorite shows?

What causes were important to you?

How do you feel about dying?

What are your favorite books?

Do you have any special talents?

Do you have any hobbies?

What is a happy memory about your parents?

What is a happy memory about your Grandparents?

Do you consider yourself religious or spiritual?

Is there a special outfit you would love to wear?

If someone can use your organs is that o.k. with you?

How do you feel about an open casket if you will
be buried?

If you are no longer able to remember what are your wishes?

If it is a huge burden to carry out your memory wishes what do you want your family to do if possible or to know?

If you are no longer able to care for yourself
what are your wishes?

If your family would like to carry out your wish about not caring for yourself but it becomes a huge burden what do you want them to know or do?

If you are in a Coma, ideally what are your wishes?

If a professional says that if you do wake you will not live a quality life or live in a vegetative state what are your wishes?

List other unique situations that you feel strongly about?

Do you wish to be buried or cremated?

What other feelings do you have about what
happens to you after you die

Is there somewhere you would like to be buried or have your ashes spread?

Do you have a will? If so where is it located?

Why did you write the will the way you did?

Did you assign anyone as power of attorney?

Do you have Bank accounts or other Insurance policies that someone needs to close?

Who else needs to be contacted when you pass away?

If you have pets, what is your wish as to how they are cared for?

If your wish is not able to be carried out on your pets, what is the back-up plan?

If the back-up pet plan does not work out what do you want your family to know?

Where were your favorite places when you were alive.

Do you have a Life Insurance Policy, and if so leave as many details as possible about how to find it here.

Why did you pick who you did for a beneficiary?

What is your wish to be done with the money?

If you have Long Term Care, Accident or Accidental Death Insurance, VA Benefits or other policies someone should know about leave the information here.

Are there any personal belongings you want to go
to a certain person and why?

Personal Belonging Information and Why? #2

Personal Belonging Information and Why? #3

Personal Belonging Information and Why? #4

Personal Belonging Information and Why? #5

Personal Belonging Information and Why? #6

Personal Belonging Information and Why? #7

Personal Belonging Information and Why? #8

If you could write your own Eulogy what would you write?

Do you have favorite Poem's, Scripture or Sayings.

favorite Poems, Scripture, or Sayings #2?

Do you have any wishes for a Headstone?

If you have a spouse what do you want them to know?

If you have Children what do you want them to know?

If you have Grandchildren what do you want them to know?

What about your final wishes is very important?

What about your final wishes is not important at all?

If someone that loves you feels bad because they are unable to say goodbye to you what do you want them to know?

If someone that loves you has other regrets related to you what do you want them to know?

If you have young children what is your wish as to what happens to them?

This next section is your chance to write a note to those you love and tell them how you feel about them. What did they mean to your life? Take this chance to let them know why they mattered to you.

1. Thank you for being a part of my life

2. Thank you for being a part of my life

3. Thank you for being a part of my life

4. Thank you for being a part of my life

5. Thank you for being a part of my life 6.
Thank you for being a part of my life

7. Thank you for being a part of my life

8. Thank you for being a part of my life

9. Thank you for being a part of my life

10. Thank you for being a part of my life

11. Thank you for being a part of my life

12. Thank you for being a part of my life

13. Thank you for being a part of my life

14. Thank you for being a part of my life

15. Thank you for being a part of my life 16.
Thank you for being a part of my life

17. Thank you for being a part of my life

18. Thank you for being a part of my life

19. Thank you for being a part of my life

20. Thank you for being a part of my life

A funny story you remember....

A funny story you remember....

A funny story you remember....

An interesting thing that happened to you?

An interesting thing that happened to you?

What else I want you to know......

What else I want you to know.....

What else I want you to know......

What else I want you to know......

www.ingramcontent.com/pod-product-compliance
Lightning Source LLC
Chambersburg PA
CBHW020554220526
45463CB00006B/2300